A true story.....written by a daughter...
reminding the world how important it is
to get your
yearly health checks!

Written By: Author Kasi Lee Freeman

Illustrated by some talented young artists
who are helping me save lives!

_____

This is _____'s HEALTH book.
(your name)

Given to me on_____.
(date)

ACKNOWLEDGEMENTS:

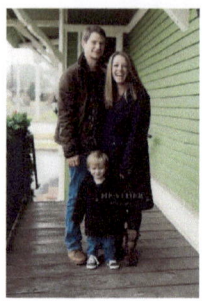

I want to thank:

#1 GOD-Thank you for showing me my purpose in life!

I will not let you down!

- My unbelievably strong mom! I couldn't have done it without you. I am so proud of you and hope that I can be as great of a mom to Sawyer as you have been to me. You are one amazing lady. I am so thankful for our relationship. Always & Forever! You are so strong! Words of the wise (you), "This too shall pass."

- My husband Nate-for everything. For not only being MY best friend, but also my dad's! For always supporting me, for you unconditional love, for enjoying spending time with my parents..and laughing at dads jokes...he loved that about you!

- My Sawyer Boy-you are my tiny angel. You keep a smile on my face. You make me proud! I love you more than you can ever imagine! You can do anything you put your mind to. Just love life! Each moment is precious! Don't ever forget that!

- Walt Alton-My counselor-God placed you in my life for so many reasons. I couldn't have done it without you...You have saved my life in so many ways..(& you made me feel less "crazy!")

- My other family and friends-too many to write here.

  Just all of my continued support! God is so great to have placed all of these amazing people in my life!

- For this book-Joyce Reed-My inspiration!

- For believing in me: Dr. Beckford-My editor & Varma Rameswar-always telling me I needed to write a book.

  - <u>**A HUGE thanks to all of my little artists:**</u>

  Addie Carruth, Rowen Walker, Ava Walker,

  Haley Jarvis & Harrison King,

  You guys ROCK! This book couldn't have happened

  without YOU!

I know everything happens for a reason,

but I do believe that some

things can be prevented.

Let me share my story and let me

hopefully save some lives!!!!

Here is my story......

THIS BOOK IS:

Intended for children, but aimed at

STUBBORN adults ←(like my dad was!)

After you have read this book,

please visit my Facebook page at:

https://www.facebook.com/pages/Is-it-time-for-your-checkup/383611915129186?sk=timeline

And please post your comments &

success stories here!

Baby Ira was born a

happy and healthy baby boy.

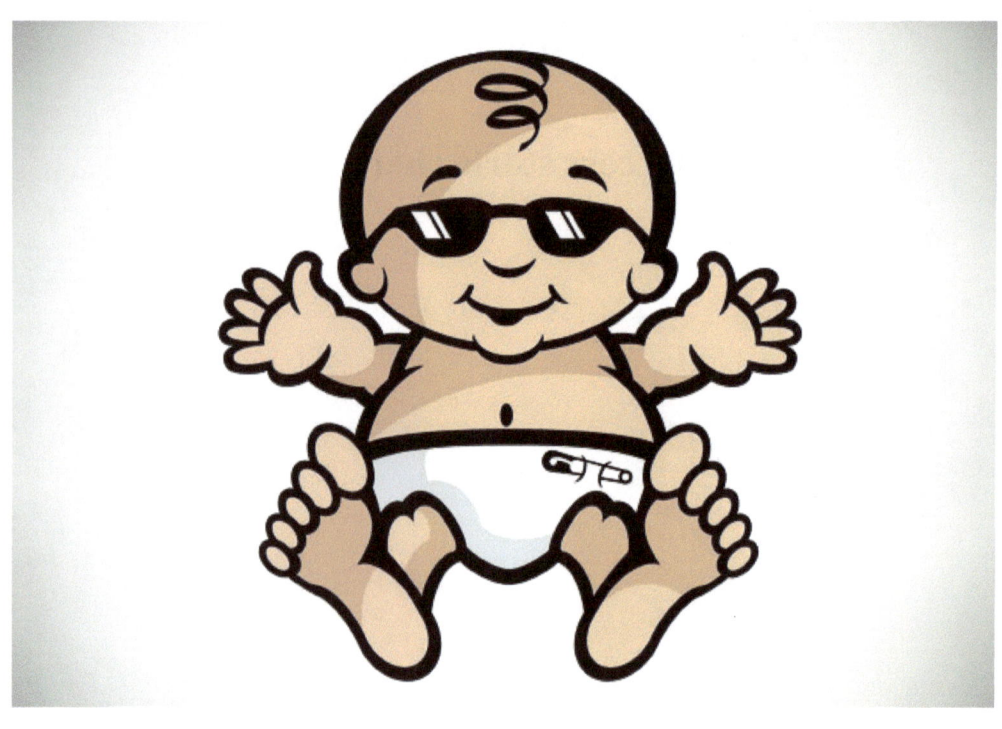

Growing up, he had <u>lots</u> of friends.

He loved to make others SMILE...

laugh...

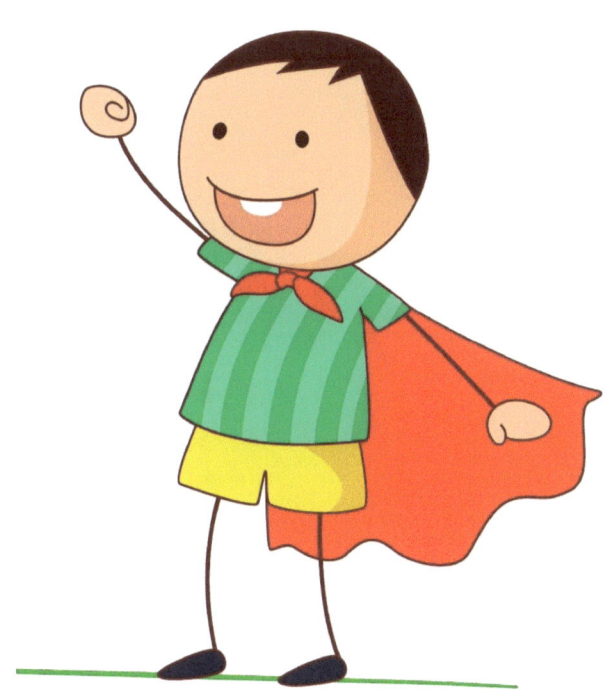

... and he told many funny jokes.

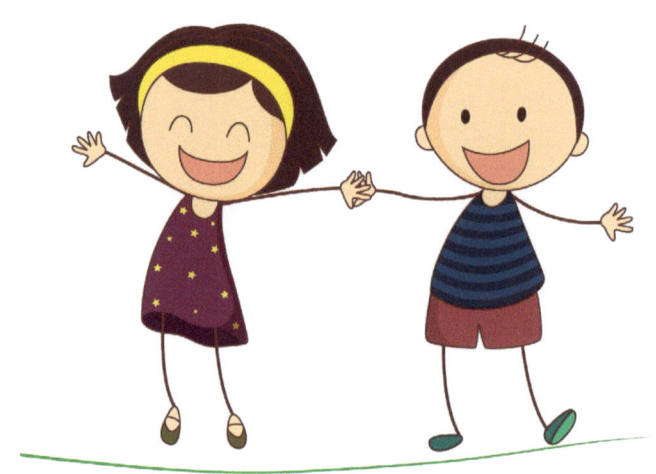

Oh, and one other thing, he had a

passion for music!

His favorite was Rock 'N' Roll!

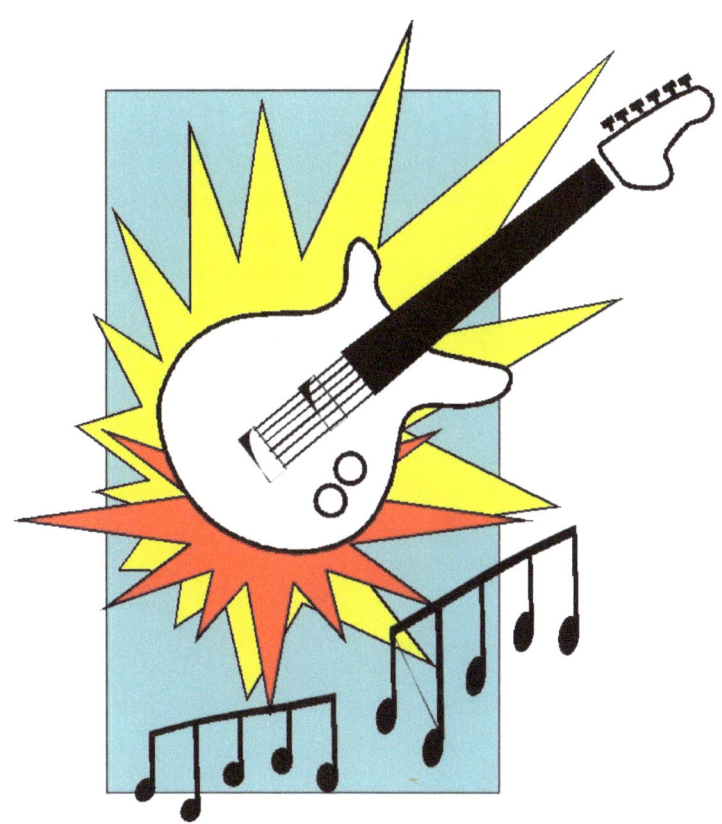

He had a mommy named Ama and a

daddy named Bubba.

He had 2 sisters and 1 brother:

Phyllis, Harriet, & Robert.

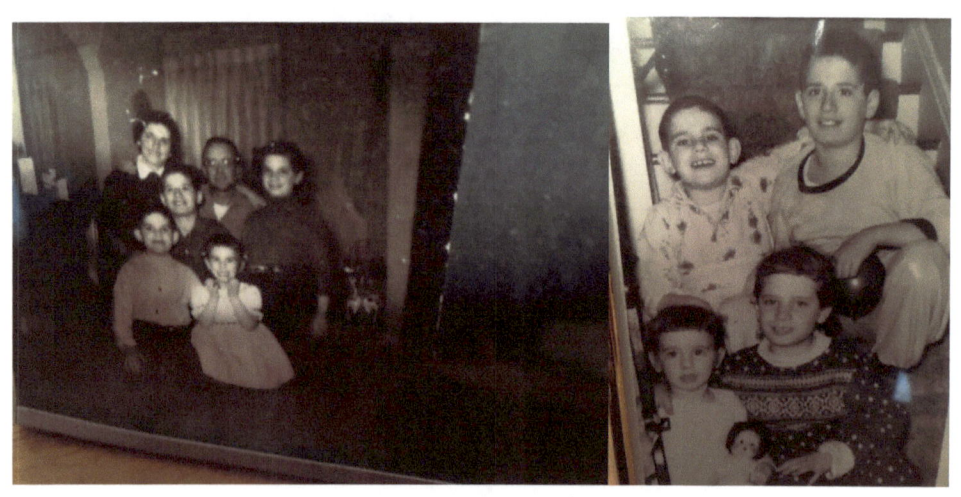

When he turned 17, he met a

beautiful woman.....Princess Debskee:

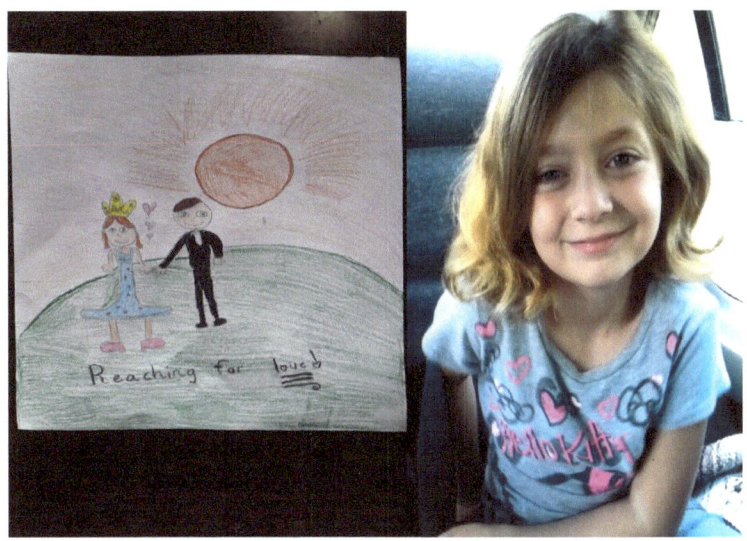

Drawing by Ava Walker: Age 9

Debskee and Ira married and decided

to have one baby girl.

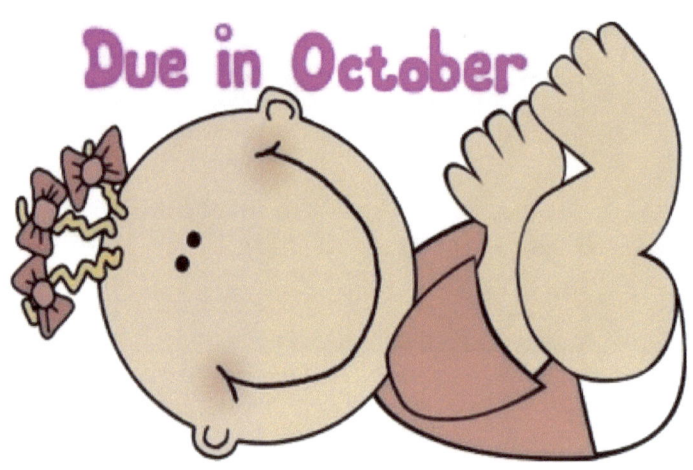

Later in life, Ira became a grandpa to a

little boy he liked to call:

"My Sawyer Boy."

This little baby was the

sunshine of his life!

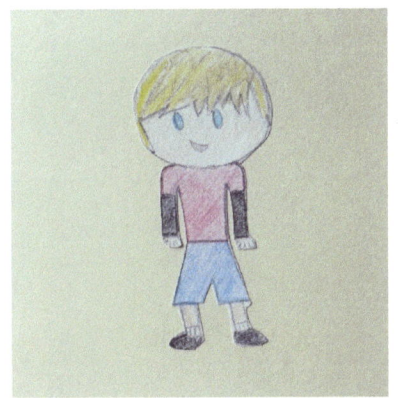 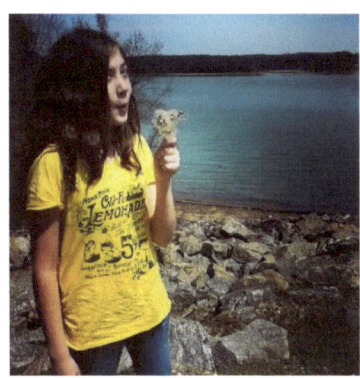

Drawing by: Rowen Walker

Ira was a silly grandpa. He loved to watch cartoons with Sawyer. He soon became known as "Poppie."

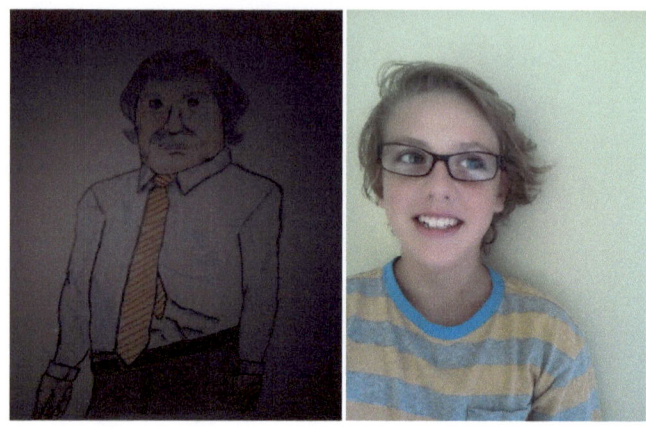

Poppie, Drawing by: Harrison King

Like most grandpas...Poppie was great at

pretty much everything!

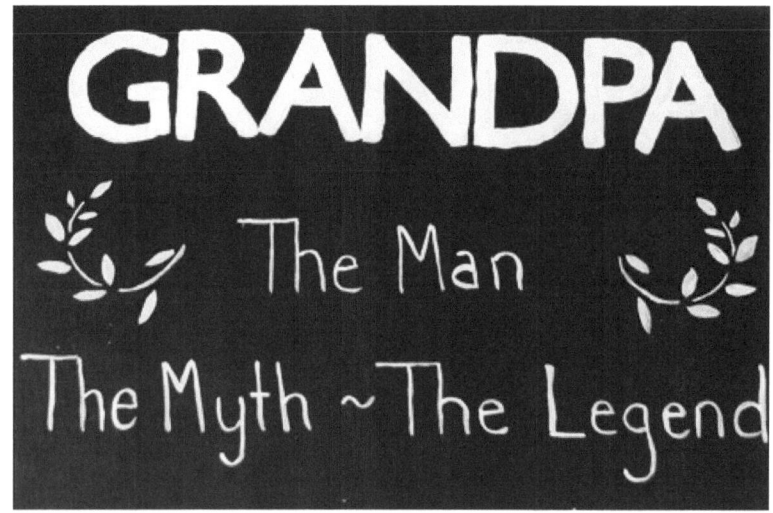

He was a dad, a brother,

a husband and a grandpa.

He decided at 60 it was time to retire.

After years and years of hard work, it was time to really start enjoying life and most of all, take time to really enjoy his grandson!

Poppie loved to travel and especially loved flying on airplanes!

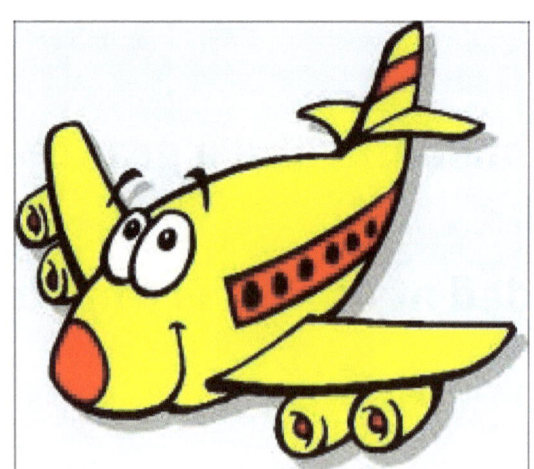

Poppie felt happy and healthy.

No one knew that Poppie hadn't been to

the doctor or dentist in <u>almost 45 years</u>.

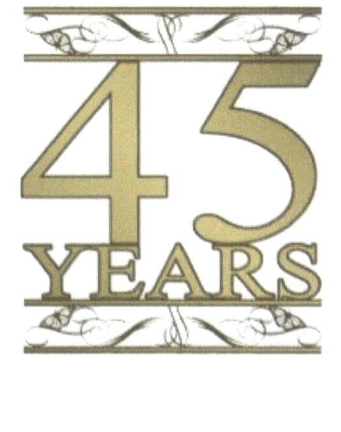

Everything seemed right in his life.

He worked hard, took care of his family,

and showed LOTS and LOTS of

love to everyone he met.

He always made you SMILE!

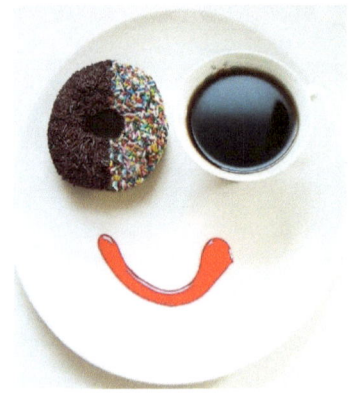

Poppie lived life to the fullest.

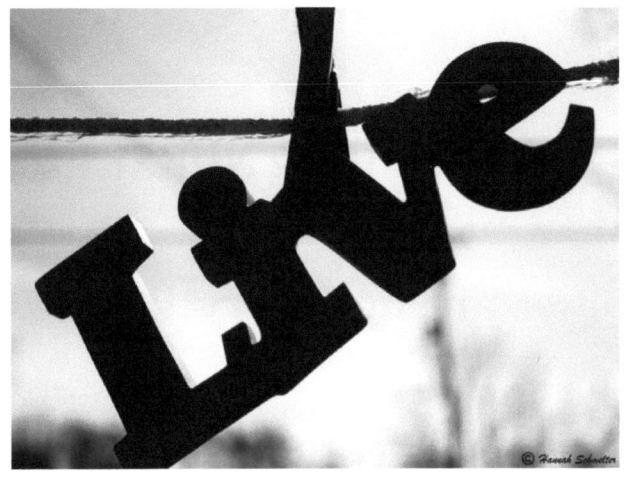

But..he forgot the <u>most important thing!</u>

He forgot to get his

yearly checkups!

Poppie needed someone to remind him

that

"DOCTORS & NURSES

are not scary!!!

They are NICE & they can <u>help</u> you!

But guess what?

Some adults are STUBBORN!

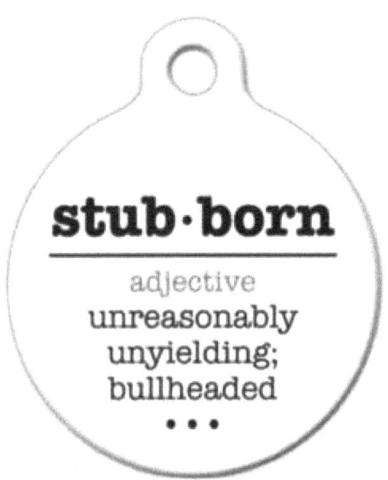

To all you beautiful children reading this story, I need you to do me a HUGE...I MEAN HUGE.....I MEAN HUMONGO, GINORMO, FAVOR!!!

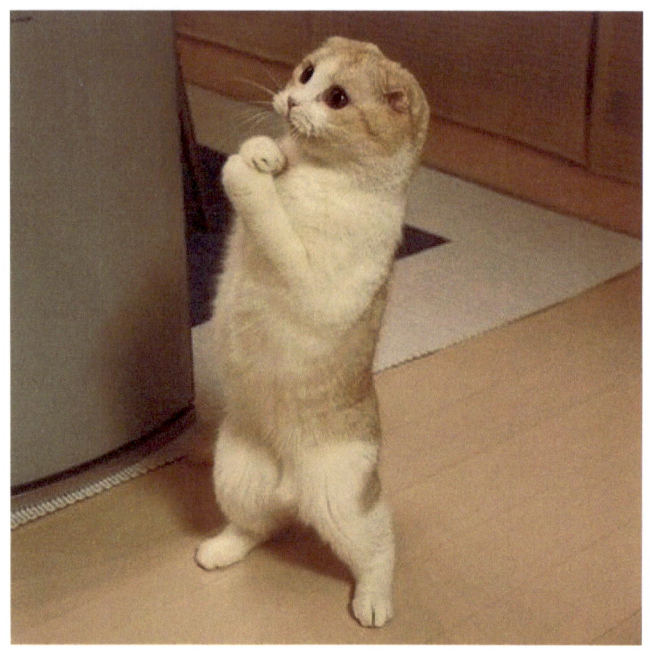

CAN YOU DO IT?

I KNOW YOU CAN!

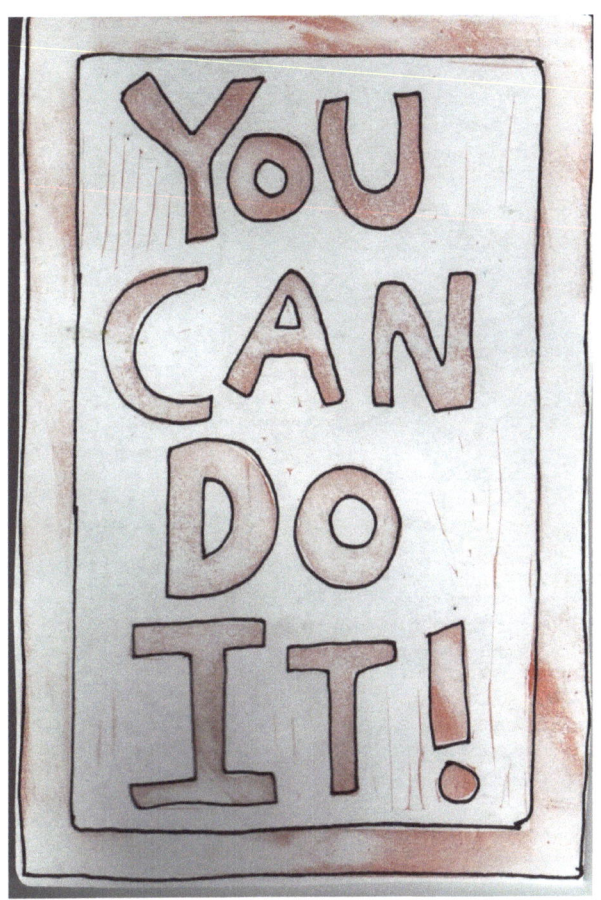

OK....

Look at your mommy or daddy, grandma

or grandpa, sister, brother, friend,

uncle..ok..

<u>anyone you love!</u>..............

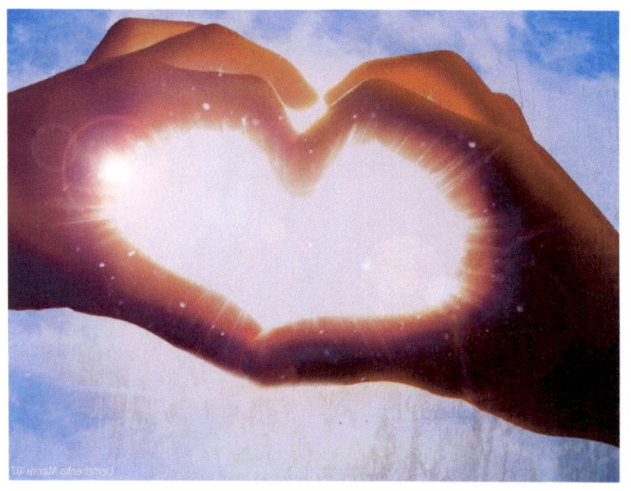

And ask them:

"Is it time for your checkup?"

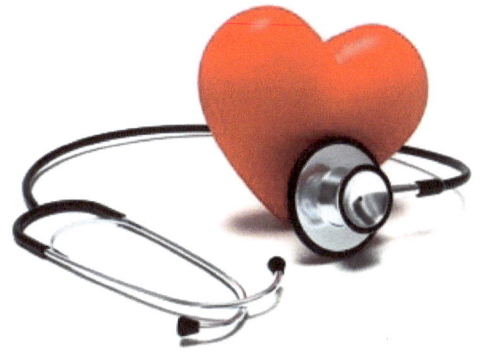

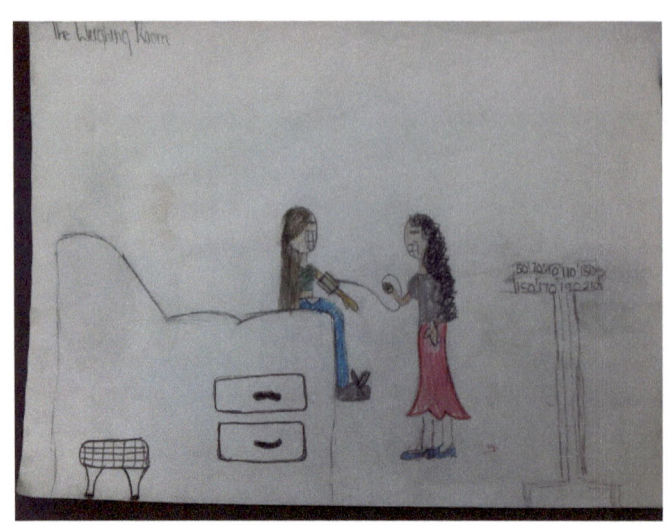

Doctor office drawings by Haley Jarvis-Age 12

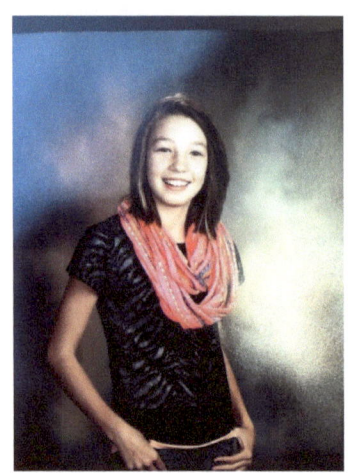

IS IT TIME FOR YOUR 6 MONTH DENTAL CHECKUP?

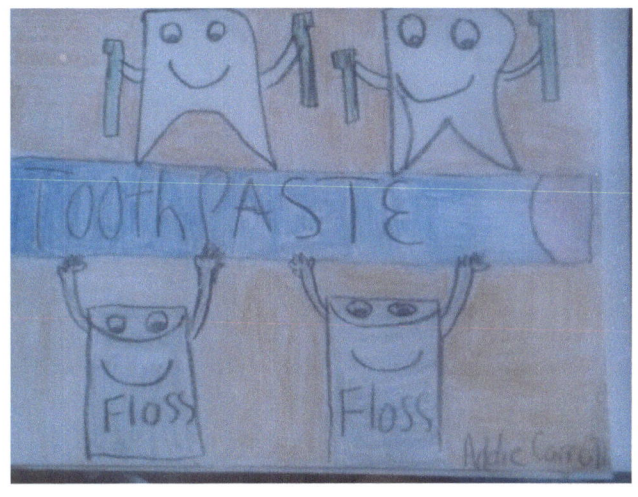

Drawing by Addie Carruth-age 9

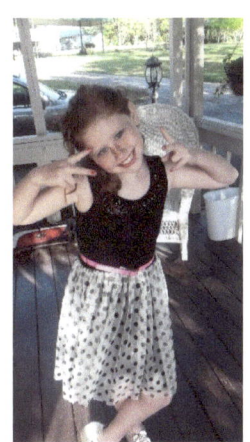

"The most important gift we give our children is unconditional love. With that as the foundation, we should nurture in them the desire to do the best they can with their God given gifts, as well as with their challenges. That way they will grow into responsible and resilient human beings that will contribute <u>positively to the world</u>."

Avril Beckford MD, FAAP,
Mother, Pediatrician, Author
Chief Pediatric Officer, WellStar Health System Past President Georgia
Chapter, Academy of Pediatrics

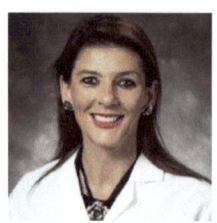

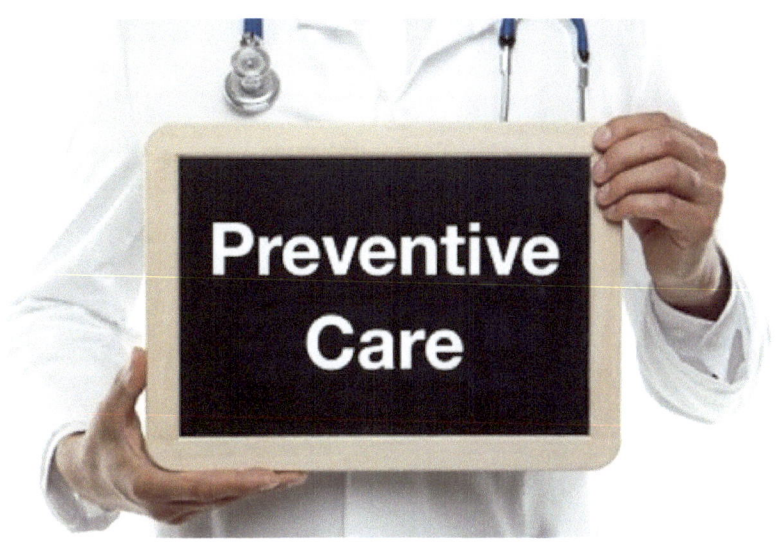

After you read this book, please fill out your own

personal health checklist:

o Date of your yearly well check:_____

o Date of your 6 month dental check up: _____

o OTHER doctor appointments:

_____

_____

_____

_____

www.ingramcontent.com/pod-product-compliance
Lightning Source LLC
Chambersburg PA
CBHW040820200526
45159CB00024B/3074